COMMON ECG RHYTHMS

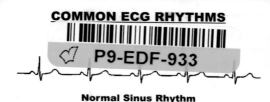

P9-EDF-933

Normal Sinus Rhythm

Ventricular Tachycardia ⚡ SHOCK ⚡

Ventricular Fibrillation ⚡ SHOCK ⚡

Premature Ventricular Contraction

Atrial Flutter

Atrial Fibrillation

MAXWELL
QUICK **MEDICAL REFERENCE**

ACLS Algorithms	**Delivery Note** **Postpartum Note** **APGAR Scoring Exam** **Estimated Delivery Date** **Glucose Tolerance Values** **Developmental Milestones** **Immunization Schedule**
Normal Lab Values **Serum Drug Levels** **Daily Body Fluids** **Ascitic / Pleural Fluids** **Helpful Equations** **Phlebotomy Tubes** **Unit Conversions**	
	History **Physical Exam**
Admit / Transfer Orders **On Service Note** **Progress Note** **Discharge Note** **Preoperative Note** **Operative Note** **Postoperative Note** **Procedure Note**	**Neurological Exam** **Mental Status Exam** **Glasgow Coma Scale** **Dermatome Maps**
	Personal Notes

6th Edition. Copyright ©2011 Robert W. Maxwell.
Published by Maxwell Publishing Company

www.MAXWELLBOOK.com

ISBN 978-0-9645191-4-5

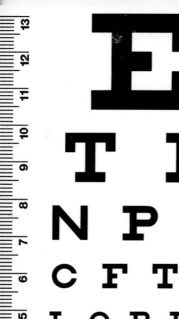

E	20/200
T L	20/100
N P D	20/70
C F T Z	20/50
L O P D E	20/40
N T F L C Z	20/30
F E Z P D T	20/25
E C T P N L	20/20

**Hold chart in good light 6 feet from eyes.
(approximately the foot of the patient's bed)
Check eyes separately with and without glasses.**

ISBN 978-0-9645191-4-5

$\frac{20}{200}$

$\frac{20}{100}$

$\frac{20}{70}$

$\frac{20}{50}$

$\frac{20}{40}$

$\frac{20}{30}$

$\frac{20}{25}$

$\frac{20}{20}$

Hold chart in good light 6 feet from eyes.
(approximately the foot of the patient's bed)
Check eyes separately with and without glasses.

DERMATOME MAP (Posterior View)

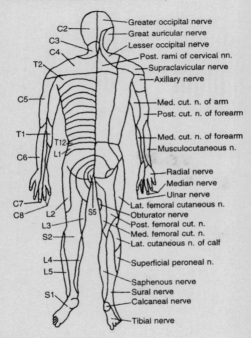

NERVE	MOTOR ACTION	SENSATION	
Obturator	Thigh adduction	Medial thigh	
Femoral	Knee extension	Anterior thigh	
Sciatic	Knee flexion	Posterolateral calf	
Peroneal	Toe extension	Dorsal foot	
Tibial	Toe flexion	Plantar foot	

ROOT	MOTOR ACTION	SENSATION	REFLEX
L1	Hip flexion (T12-L3)	Below inguinal ligament	--
L2	Hip adduction (L2-L4)	Middle thigh	--
L3	Knee extension (L2-L4)	Lower thigh	--
L4	Foot dorsiflexion / inversion	Medial leg, medial foot	Patellar
L5	Toe extension	Lateral leg, dorsal foot	--
S1	Foot plantar flexion / eversion	Lateral foot	Achilles

DERMATOME MAP (Anterior View)

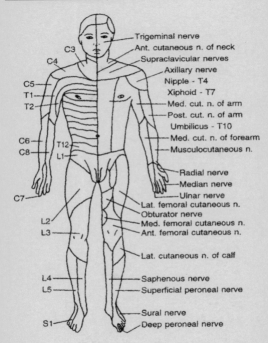

NERVE	MOTOR ACTION	SENSATION
Axillary	Shoulder abduction	Lateral shoulder
Musculocutaneous	Elbow flexion	Lateral forearm
Median	Thumb opposition	Lateral palm
Radial	Finger extension	Dorsolateral hand
Ulnar	Finger ab/adduction	Medial hand

ROOT	MOTOR ACTION	SENSATION	REFLEX
C5	Shoulder abduction	Lateral arm	Biceps
C6	Wrist extension	Thumb, index finger	Brachioradialis
C7	Wrist flexion	Middle finger	Triceps
C8	Finger flexion	Ring, small finger	--
T1	Finger ab/adduction	Medial arm	--

MENTAL STATUS EXAM (FOLSTEIN)

Maximum
Score

5   What time is it? (year, season, month, day, date)

5   Where are we? (state, county, town, hospital, floor)

3   Test giver names 3 objects, 1 second to say each. Ask patient to repeat all 3. Give 1 point for each correct answer. Repeat 3 objects until patient learns them. Note number of trials to learn.

5   Serial 7's from 100 to 5 answers (93,86,79,72,65) or spell "world" backwards.

3   Ask for 3 objects named above.

2   Test giver points to pencil and watch and patient names them.

1   Repeat the following: "No ifs, ands or buts."

3   Follow 3 step command: "Take the paper in your right hand, fold it in half, and put it on the floor."

1   Read and obey the following: CLOSE YOUR EYES.

1   Write a sentence.

1   Copy design.

     Assess level of consciousness along a continuum:
     ALERT -- DROWSY -- STUPOR -- COMA

NOTE: Scoring exam used to evaluate and follow a patient's mental state.
Score is sum of the eleven evaluations. Range 0 (worst) to 30 (best). Good > 20.

GLASGOW COMA SCALE

EYE RESPONSE (E)
4 = Open spontaneously   2 = Open to pain
3 = Open to verbal command   1 = No response

VERBAL RESPONSE (V)
5 = Oriented, converses   2 = Incomprehensible sounds
4 = Disoriented, converses   1 = No response
3 = Inappropriate responses

MOTOR RESPONSE (M)
6 = Obeys verbal command   3 = Decorticate (flex) to pain
5 = Localizes to pain   2 = Decerebrate (extend) to pain
4 = Withdrawal from pain   1 = No response to pain

NOTE: Scoring exam used to monitor changes in level of consciousness.
Score is sum of eye, verbal, and motor responses. Range 3 (worst) to 15 (normal).

NEUROLOGICAL EXAM

MENTAL STATUS EXAM (see other side)

CRANIAL NERVES
I, **OLFACTORY** – smell
II, **OPTIC** – visual acuity / fields and fundoscopic exam of each eye
III, IV, VI; **OCULOMOTOR, TROCHLEAR, ABDUCENS** – eyelid opening; extraocular movements (IV, superior oblique; VI, lateral rectus; III, all others); direct and consensual pupillary light reflexes
V, **TRIGEMINAL** (V1, ophthalmic; V2, maxillary; V3, mandibular) – corneal reflex, facial sensation, jaw opening, bite strength
VII, **FACIAL** – eyebrow raise, eyelid close, smile, frown, pucker, taste
VIII, **VESTIBULOCOCHLEAR** – auditory acuity of each ear, Rinne (air v. bone conduction) and Weber (lateralizing) tests, oculocephalic reflex (doll's eye maneuver), oculovestibular reflex (ear canal caloric stimulation)
IX, X; **GLOSSOPHARYNGEAL, VAGUS** – palate elevation, swallowing, posterior taste, phonation, gag reflex
XI, **SPINAL ACCESSORY** – lateral head rotation, neck flexion, shoulder shrug
XII, **HYPOGLOSSAL** – tongue protrusion and strength on lateral deviation

SENSATION
Test and contralaterally compare pain / temperature, vibratory, and proprioceptive (Romberg test, joint position) sensation; stereognosis; graphasthesia; and two point discrimination.

STRENGTH
Test and contralaterally compare extremity muscle groups listed with the dermatome maps.
Grading: 5/5 - Movement against gravity with full resistance
             4/5 - Movement against gravity with some resistance
             3/5 - Movement against gravity only
             2/5 - Movement with gravity eliminated
             1/5 - Visible / palpable muscle contraction but no movement
             0/5 - No contraction

REFLEXES
Test and contralaterally compare triceps (C7, radial n.), biceps (C5, musculocutaneous n.), brachioradialis (C6, radial n.), patellar (L4, femoral n.), Achilles (S1, tibial n.) and Babinski sign.
Grading: 4+ - Hyperactive with clonus
             3+ - Hyperactive
             2+ - Normal
             1+ - Hypoactive
             0 - No reflex

CEREBELLUM
Test finger-to-nose, heel-to-shin, and rapid alternating hand movements.

GAIT
Test tandem gait, walking on heels and toes.

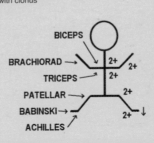

BICEPS
BRACHIORAD →   2+   2+
TRICEPS → 2+
PATELLAR → 2+
BABINSKI → 2+ ↓
ACHILLES →

HISTORY AND PHYSICAL EXAM

REVIEW OF SYSTEMS (continued)

GENITAL: male: penile discharge or sores, testicular pain or masses, hernias; **female:** menarche, period regularity, frequency, duration, dysmenorrhea, last period, itching, discharge, sores, pregnancies and complications, miscarriages / abortions, birth control, menopause, hot flashes / sweats; **general:** STD history / treatment; sex interest, function, problems, contraception methods

VASCULAR: leg edema, claudication, varicose veins, thromboses / emboli

MUSCULOSKELETAL: muscle weakness, pain; joint stiffness, range of motion, instability, redness, swelling, arthritis, gout

NEUROLOGIC: loss of sensation / numbness, tingling, tremors, weakness / paralysis, fainting / blackouts, seizures

HEMATOLOGIC: anemia, easy bruising / bleeding, petechiae, purpura, transfusions

ENDOCRINE: heat / cold intolerance, excessive sweating, polyuria, polydipsia, polyphagia, thyroid problems, diabetes

PSYCHIATRIC: mood, anxiety, depression, tension, memory

PHYSICAL EXAM:

GENERAL: sex, race, state of health, stature, development, dress, hygiene, affect

VITALS: blood pressure, pulse, respirations, temperature, height, weight

SKIN: skin scars, rashes, bruises, tattoos; hair consistency; nail pitting, stippling

HEAD: size, shape, trauma

EYES: pupil size, shape, reactivity; conjunctival injection; scleral icterus; fundal papilledema, hemorrhage; lids; extraocular movements; visual fields and acuity

EARS: shape / symmetry, tenderness, discharge, external canal / tympanic membrane inflammation, gross auditory acuity

NOSE: symmetry, tenderness, discharge, mucosa / turbinate inflammation, frontal / maxillary sinus tenderness

MOUTH, THROAT: hygiene, dentures, erythema, exudate, tonsillar enlargement

NECK: masses, range of motion, spine / trachea deviation, thyroid size / masses

BREASTS: skin changes, symmetry, tenderness, masses, dimpling, discharge

HEART: rate, rhythm, murmurs, rubs, gallops, clicks, precordial movements

LUNGS: chest symmetry with respirations, wheezes, crackles, vocal fremitus, whispered pectoriloquy, percussion, diaphragmatic excursion

ABDOMEN: shape, scars, bowel sounds, consistency (soft / firm), tenderness, rebound, masses, guarding, spleen size / liver span, percussion (tympany, shifting dullness), costovertebral angle (CVA) tenderness

GENITOURINARY: male: rashes, ulcers, scars, nodules, induration, discharge, scrotal masses, hernias; **female:** external genitalia, vaginal mucosa, and cervix: inflammation, discharge, bleeding, ulcers, nodules, masses; internal vaginal support; bimanual and rectovaginal palpation of cervix, uterus, ovaries

RECTAL: sphincter tone, prostate consistency, masses, occult stool blood

MUSCULOSKELETAL: muscle atrophy, weakness; joint range of motion, instability, redness, swelling, tenderness; spine deviation; gait

VASCULAR: carotid, radial, femoral, popliteal, posterior tibial, dorsalis pedis pulses; carotid bruits, jugular venous distension, edema, varicose veins

LYMPHATIC: cervical, supra/infraclavicular, axillary, trochlear, inguinal adenopathy

NEUROLOGIC: cranial nerves, sensation, strength, reflexes, cerebellum, gait

LABS

hematology, chemistry, urinalysis, cultures, ECG, x-rays, CT/MRI scan, etc.

ASSESSMENT / PLAN

differential diagnosis, supporting history and exam; medication changes, lab tests, procedures, consults, etc.

HISTORY AND PHYSICAL EXAM

CHIEF COMPLAINT (health problem / complaint in patient's own words)

HISTORY OF PRESENT ILLNESS
chronological order of time / place of symptom(s) onset, duration, frequency, location, quality, quantity / severity, aggravating / alleviating factors, associated symptoms, self treatment, relevant laboratory values, pertinent negatives

PAST MEDICAL HISTORY
GENERAL HEALTH; date, type, outcome, complications of **CHILDHOOD ILLNESSES** (measles, mumps, rubella, whooping cough, chicken pox, rheumatic fever, scarlet fever, polio); **ADULT ILLNESSES; ACCIDENTS / INJURIES**; hospitalizations not already listed; **IMMUNIZATIONS** (DPT, MMR, polio, hepatitis B, H. influenza, S. pneumoniae, varicella); **SCREENING TESTS** (hematocrit, urinalysis, tuberculin skin test, pap smear, mammogram, occult stool blood, cholesterol)

PAST SURGICAL HISTORY
operation date, type, reason, outcome, blood transfusions, complications

FAMILY HISTORY
age, health / death of parents, siblings, spouse, children; **CHECK** diabetes, heart disease, hypertension, stroke, cancer, bleeding disorders, asthma, arthritis, tuberculosis, epilepsy, mental illness, symptoms of presenting illness

SOCIAL HISTORY
birthplace, education, employment, religion, marriage / divorce, living accommodations, persons at home, diet, exercise, hobbies

MEDICATIONS
name, dose, frequency, duration, reason for taking, compliance, availability

ALLERGIES
medications / substances causing reactions (rash, swelling, difficulty breathing, etc.)

TOBACCO, ALCOHOL, DRUGS
type, amount, frequency, duration, reactions, treatment

REVIEW OF SYSTEMS
GENERAL: weight change, fatigue, weakness, fever, chills, night sweats
SKIN: skin, hair, nail changes; itching; rashes; sores; lumps; moles
HEAD: trauma; headache location, frequency, nausea, vomiting, visual changes
EYES: glasses, contact lenses, blurriness, tearing, itching, acute visual loss
EARS: hearing loss, tinnitus, vertigo, discharge, earache
NOSE, SINUSES: rhinorrhea, stuffiness, sneezing, itching, allergy, epistaxis
MOUTH, THROAT, NECK: bleeding gums, hoarseness, sore throat, swollen neck
BREASTS: skin changes, masses / lumps, pain, discharge, self exams
CARDIAC: hypertension, murmurs, angina, palpitations, dyspnea on exertion, orthopnea, paroxysmal nocturnal dyspnea, edema, last ECG
RESPIRATORY: shortness of breath, wheeze, cough, sputum, hemoptysis, pneumonia, asthma, bronchitis, emphysema, tuberculosis, last chest X-ray
GI: appetite, nausea, vomiting, indigestion, dysphagia, bowel movement frequency / change, stool color, diarrhea, constipation, bleeding (hemetemesis, hemorrhoids, melena or hematechezia), abdominal pain, jaundice, hepatitis
URINARY: frequency, hesitancy, urgency, polyuria, dysuria, hematuria, nocturia, incontinence, stones, infection

ESTIMATED DELIVERY DATE (NAEGELE'S RULE)

First day of last normal menstrual period: August 11, 2011 (example)

1. Add 7 days. (11th becomes 18th)
2. Subtract 3 months. (August becomes May)
3. Add 1 year. (2011 becomes 2012)

Estimated Delivery Date: May 18, 2012

GLUCOSE TOLERANCE VALUES

ADULT NONPREGNANT (75g PO)

Diabetes Mellitus:
A1C ≥ 6.5% or
Fasting Glucose ≥ 126 mg/dL or
2 Hour OGTT ≥ 200 mg/dL or
Random Glucose ≥ 200 mg/dL and sx

A1C = ESTIMATED AVG GLUCOSE (eAG)

6% = 126 mg/dL	8.5% = 197 mg/dL
6.5% = 140 mg/dL	9% = 212 mg/dL
7% = 154 mg/dL	9.5% = 226 mg/dL
7.5% = 169 mg/dL	10% = 240 mg/dL
8% = 183 mg/dL	eAG=(28.7xA1C)−46.7

ADULT PREGNANT (24-28 weeks)

1 hour: 140 mg/dL   (50g PO)

Perform 3 hour oral glucose tolerance test (OGTT) if 140 mg/dL is exceeded.

Fasting: 95 mg/dL (100g PO)
1 hour: 180 mg/dL
2 hours: 155 mg/dL
3 hours: 140 mg/dL

Gestational Diabetes:
Two or more values are exceeded.

DEVELOPMENTAL MILESTONES

AGE	ABILITY
2 mos	smile, follow past midline, ooo/aah, head up 45°
4 mos	regard hand, grasp rattle, squeal/laugh, bear weight on legs
6 mos	feed self, reach, imitate speech sounds, pull to sit-no head lag
9 mos	take 2 cubes, jabber, pull to stand, sit unsupported
12 mos	wave bye, pat-a-cake, pincer grasp, dada/mama, stand 2 sec.
15 mos	play ball with examiner, scribbles, 2 words, walk well
18 mos	use spoon/fork, drink from cup, 2 cube tower, 3 words, runs
24 mos	remove garment, 4 cube tower, 6 body parts, walk up steps
3 yrs	wash/dry hands, 8 cube tower, 2 adjectives, broad jump
4 yrs	dress-no help, copy circle, speech all understandable, hops

IMMUNIZATION SCHEDULE

BIRTH: HepB
2 MONTHS: HepB, RV, DTaP, Hib, PCV, IPV
4 MONTHS: RV, DTaP, Hib, PCV, IPV
6 MONTHS: HepB, RV, DTaP, Hib, PCV, IPV, Influenza (yearly)
12-15 MONTHS: DTaP, Hib, PCV, MMR, Varicella, HepA (2 doses >6 mos apart)
4-6 YEARS: DTaP, IPV, MMR, Varicella

NOTE: See complete CDC recommendations (cdc.gov) and prescribing information before administration. HepB = hepatitis B. RV = rotavirus. DTaP = diphtheria tetanus acellular pertussis. Hib = Haemophilus influenzae type B. PCV = Pneumococcal vaccine. IPV = Inactivated polio vaccine. MMR = measles mumps rubella. HepA = hepatitis A.

DELIVERY NOTE

DELIVERY DATE/TIME:
PHYSICIANS: attending, residents, students who scrubbed
MOTHER: age, race, gravida x, para x, group B strep positive/negative
ANESTHESIA: epidural, pudendal, local, none
DELIVERY: spontaneous vaginal, low transverse C-section, classical C-section
INFANT: male / female, weight, APGAR 1 & 5 min, bulb / DeLee suction
UMBILICAL CORD: 2 or 3 vessel, nuchal cord, blood sent to lab
PLACENTA: delivery time/method, intact, fragmented, meconium stained
MEDS: amount in cc of carboprost, methylergonovine, oxytocin, etc.
CLOSURE: episiotomy, nth degree laceration, uterus/abdominal incision with xx suture
ESTIMATED BLOOD LOSS: amount in cc
COMPLICATIONS:
CONDITION: of mother and infant

POSTPARTUM NOTE

S: patient comments or complaints, nursing comments, **CHECK** pain control, breast erythema/tenderness, quantity/trend of vaginal bleeding, urination, flatus, bowel movement, lower extremity swelling, ambulation, breast or bottle feed, birth control type
O: VITALS: blood pressure, pulse, respirations, temperature
  INS/OUTS: IV fluid, PO intake, emesis, urine, stool
  EXAM: breath sounds, bowel sounds, fundal height / consistency, incision / episiotomy condition, lower extremity edema, Homan's sign
  MEDS: RhoGAM, pain med, iron, vitamins, laxative, contraception
  LABS: CBC, Rh status, rubella status
A: assessments based on data above
P: medications, lab tests, rubella immunization, consults, discharge

APGAR SCORING EXAM

APPEARANCE
2 = Entire body pink
1 = Pink body with blue extremities
0 = Entire body blue or pale

PULSE
2 = >100 beats/minute
1 = <100 beats/minute
0 = Absent

GRIMACE
2 = Cough, sneeze, or vigorous cry
1 = Grimace or slight cry
0 = No response

ACTIVITY
2 = Active movement
1 = Some movement
0 = Limp, motionless

RESPIRATIONS
2 = Strong, crying
1 = Slow, irregular
0 = Absent

NOTE: Scoring exam for condition of newborn infants. Determined at 1 and 5 minutes after birth. Score is sum of five assessments. Range 0 (worst) to 10 (best). Score ≥7 good; 4-6 assist, stimulate; <4 resuscitate.

PREOPERATIVE NOTE

PRE-OP DIAGNOSIS:
PROCEDURE: planned surgery
LABS: CBC, chemistries, PT/PTT, urinalysis, etc.
CHEST X-RAY: note findings
EKG: note findings
BLOOD: not needed, type/screen or type/cross 2 units packed RBCs, etc.
ORDERS: NPO, preoperative antibiotics, skin or colon preps, etc.
PERMIT: Signed and on chart. (if so)

OPERATIVE NOTE

PRE-OP DIAGNOSIS:
POST-OP DIAGNOSIS:
PROCEDURE: surgery performed
SURGEONS: attending, residents, students who scrubbed
FINDINGS: acutely inflamed gallbladder, sigmoid colon mass, etc.
ANESTHESIA: general endotracheal (GETA), spinal, local, etc.
FLUIDS: amount and type (electrolytes, blood, etc. in cc or units)
ESTIMATED BLOOD LOSS: amount in cc
DRAINS: type and location (T-tube in RUQ)
SPECIMENS: type sent to pathology (gallbladder and cystic duct, etc.)
COMPLICATIONS:
CONDITION: stable, extubated, transferred to recovery room, etc.

POSTOPERATIVE NOTE

PROCEDURE: surgery performed
S: patient comments or complaints, nursing comments, **CHECK**
consciousness (alert, oriented, drowsy), pain control, etc.
O: VITALS: blood pressure, pulse, respirations, temp, oxygen sat, etc.
  INS/OUTS: IV fluid, PO intake, emesis, urine, stool, drains, etc.
  EXAM: physical findings (incision/dressing, neurovascular status, etc.)
  MEDS: routine or new medications (antibiotics, DVT prophylaxis, etc.)
  LABS: results of any since surgery
A: assessments based on data above
P: medication changes, lab tests, procedures, consults, discharge, etc.

PROCEDURE NOTE

PROCEDURE:
PERMIT: Procedure, benefits, risks (include those of bleeding,
infection, injury, anesthesia, and allergic reaction), and alternatives
explained to the patient who voiced understanding of the information.
Their questions were sought and answered. Patient agreed to proceed
with the (spinal tap, paracentesis, etc.) Permit signed and on chart. (if so)
INDICATION: suspected meningitis, ascites, etc.
PHYSICIAN(S):
DESCRIPTION: Area prepped and draped in a sterile fashion. (Local,
spinal, etc.) anesthetic administered with (cc medication). Describe
technique including instruments, body location, occurrences, etc.
COMPLICATIONS:
ESTIMATED BLOOD LOSS: amount in cc
DISPOSITION: Pt. alert, oriented, and resting; breathing nonlabored;
extremities neurovascularly intact; incision clean, dry and intact; etc.

ADMIT / TRANSFER ORDERS

ADMIT / TRANSFER: floor, room, service, attending, residents
DIAGNOSIS: list in order of priority
CONDITION: good, stable, fair, guarded, critical, etc.
VITALS: q4', q shift, routine
ACTIVITY: ad lib, bed rest, up to chair, ambulate three times a day, etc.
DIET: regular, ADA (diabetic), low sodium, clear liquid, NPO, etc.
INS AND OUTS: strict, routine, ad lib, etc.
  IV FLUIDS: D5NS to run at 120 mL/hr, etc.
  DRAINS: Foley to gravity, nasogastric tube to intermittent suction, etc.
MEDS: antibiotics, anticoagulants, antiemetics, insulin, O_2, pain meds, etc.
ALLERGIES: specific medications / substances, NKDA, etc.
LABS: CBC, chemistries, X-rays, MRI/CT, EKG, pulse oximetry, etc.
MONITORS: arterial line, noninvasive BP, CVP, pulse ox, telemetry, etc.
RESPIRATORY CARE: updrafts, endotracheal suctioning, spirometry, etc.
DRESSING CARE: dressing changes, DVT stockings, etc.
HOUSE OFFICER CALLS: Notify H.O. if BP>150/100, temp>101°F, etc.

ON SERVICE NOTE

ADMIT DATE:
ADMIT DIAGNOSIS: list in order of importance
HOSPITAL COURSE: changes over time, lab studies, procedures, results
PHYSICAL EXAM: brief, targeted
PROBLEM LIST: list in order of importance
ASSESSMENT: based on above data
PLAN: medication changes, lab tests, procedures, consults, etc.

PROGRESS NOTE (SOAP Note)

S: patient comments or complaints, nursing comments
O: VITALS: blood pressure, pulse, respirations, temp, weight, O_2 sat
  INS/OUTS: IV fluid, PO intake, emesis, urine, stool, drains
  EXAM: physical findings
  MEDS: pertinent routine or new medications
  LABS: new laboratory or procedure results
A: assessments based on data above
P: medication changes, lab tests, procedures, consults, discharge

DISCHARGE NOTE

ADMISSION / DISCHARGE DATES:
ADMISSION / DISCHARGE DIAGNOSES:
SERVICE: service name, attending, residents
REFERRING PHYSICIAN:
CONSULTS: physicians, services, dates
PROCEDURES: dates of surgery, lumbar punctures, angiograms, etc.
HISTORY, PHYSICAL EXAM: pertinent admission H & P and lab tests
COURSE: summary of treatment and progress during hospital stay
DISCHARGE CONDITION: good, stable, fair, guarded, critical, etc.
DISPOSITION: discharged to home, specific nursing home, etc.
MEDICATIONS: discharge meds with dosage, administration, refills
INSTRUCTIONS: activity restrictions, diet, dressing and/or cast care,
  symptoms to warrant further treatment, etc.
FOLLOW-UP: follow-up appointment, emergency phone number, etc.

HELPFUL EQUATIONS

ANION GAP: $Na - (Cl + HCO_3)$

FRACTIONAL Na EXCRETION:

$$\frac{\text{urine Na} \times \text{serum creatinine}}{\text{serum Na} \times \text{urine creatinine}}$$

MAINTENANCE HOURLY FLUIDS:

4 mL for each kg 1-10 +
2 mL for each kg 11-30 +
1 mL for each kg > 30

ex: 70 kg person: 120 mL/hr

CORRECTED Na:

$Na + [(\text{glucose} - 100) \times 0.016]$

Aa GRADIENT:

$[(713 \times FIO_2) - (PaCO_2 / 0.8)] - PaO_2$

ARTERIAL BLOOD GAS RULE:

Δ 10 mm Hg $PaCO_2 = \Delta$ 0.08 pH

OSMOLALITY: $2 \times Na + \text{glucose}/18 + BUN/2.8$

BODY WATER DEFICIT: (liters)

$$\frac{0.6 \times \text{weight (kg)} \times (\text{patient Na} - \text{normal Na})}{\text{normal Na}}$$

CREATININE CLEARANCE: (estimate of GFR)

$$\frac{\text{urine creatinine} \times \text{urine volume (mL)}}{\text{serum creatinine} \times \text{time (min)}}$$

$$\frac{(140 - \text{age}) \times \text{weight (kg)} \ (\times 0.85 \text{ for females})}{72 \times \text{serum creatinine (mg/dL)}}$$

CORRECTED TOTAL Ca:

$[0.8 \times (\text{normal albumin} - \text{patient albumin})] + Ca$

MEAN ARTERIAL PRESSURE:

diastolic BP + [(systolic BP − diastolic BP) / 3]

BODY SURFACE AREA: (m²)

$\sqrt{\text{height (cm)} \times \text{weight (kg)} / 3600}$

PHLEBOTOMY TUBES

COLOR	USES
Red	Chemistries, amylase, ANA, CEA, complement, Coombs, C-peptide, CPK isoenzymes, cross-match, folate, glucose tolerance, hepatitis, HIV, IgA, IgD, IgG, IgM, iron, lipase, methemoglobin, most drug levels, PSA, RPR/VDRL, thyroid
Yellow	Blood cultures
Green	Ammonia, chromosome and HLA analysis, thiamine
Blue	PT, PTT, INR, factor assays, fibrinogen, fibrin split products
Purple	CBC, ABO type, cortisol, ESR, helper T-cell, renin (on ice)
Gray	Ethanol, lactate (on ice), sulfa levels

UNIT CONVERSIONS

36.0°C = 96.8°F

1 in = 2.54 cm	1 cm = 0.3937 in	37.0 °C = 98.6 °F
1 ft = 0.3048 m	1 m = 3.2808 ft	37.8 °C = 100.0 °F
1 mi = 1.6093 km	1 km = 0.6214 mi	38.0 °C = 100.4 °F
		38.3 °C = 101.0 °F
1 fl oz = 29.573 mL	1 mL = 0.033841 fl oz	38.9 °C = 102.0 °F
1 qt = 0.94633 L	1 L = 1.0567 qt	39.0 °C = 102.2 °F
1 gal = 3.7854 L	1 L = 0.26417 gal	39.4 °C = 103.0 °F
1 teaspoon = 5 mL	1 tablespoon = 15 mL	40.0 °C = 104.0 °F
1 oz = 28.350 g	1 g = 0.035274 oz	°F = (°C × 9/5) + 32
1 lb = 0.45359 kg	1 kg = 2.2046 lbs	°C = (°F − 32) × 5/9

SERUM DRUG LEVELS*

DRUG	THERAPEUTIC	TOXIC
Carbamazepine (Tegretol)	4-12 µg/mL	>12 µg/mL
Digoxin (Lanoxin)	0.8-2.0 ng/mL	>2.0 ng/mL
Ethosuximide (Zarontin)	40-100 µg/mL	>150 µg/mL
Lidocaine (Xylocaine)	1.5-6 µg/mL	>6 µg/mL
Lithium (Eskalith)	0.6-1.2 mEq/L	>1.5 mEq/L
NAPA (N-acetyl procainamide)	5-30 µg/mL	>40 µg/mL
Phenobarbital	15-40 µg/mL	>35 µg/mL
Phenytoin (Dilantin)	10-20 µg/mL	>20 µg/mL
Procainamide (Procan)	3-10 µg/mL	>10 µg/mL
Quinidine (Quinaglute)	1.5-5 µg/mL	>5 µg/mL
Theophylline (Theo-Dur)	10-20 µg/mL	>20 µg/mL
Valproic Acid (Depakene)	50-100 µg/mL	>100 µg/mL

DRUG	PEAK	TROUGH
Amikacin (Amikin)	25-35 µg/mL	<10 µg/mL
Gentamicin (Garamycin)	4-6 µg/mL	<2 µg/mL
Tobramycin (Nebcin)	4-6 µg/mL	<2 µg/mL
Vancomycin (Vancocin)	20-40 µg/mL	<10 µg/mL

*NOTE: Values for adults. See complete prescribing information before treatment. Monitor closely for signs / symptoms of drug toxicity. Do not base treatment on drug levels alone.

DAILY BODY FLUIDS

	mEq/L				VOLUME
FLUID	Na	K	Cl	HCO$_3$	(mL/day)
Biliary	145	5	100	**35**	50-800
Diarrheal	60	**35**	40	**30**	varies
Gastric	60	**10**	**130**	0	100-4000
Ileal	130	5	100	**50**	100-9000
Pancreatic	140	5	75	**115**	100-800
Salivary	10	**26**	10	**30**	500-2000

ASCITIC / PLEURAL FLUIDS

FLUID	S.G.	PROTEIN	LDH	PROTEIN (fluid:serum)	LDH (fluid:serum)
Transudate	< 1.016	< 3.0 g/dL	< 200 U/L	< 0.5	< 0.6
Exudate	> 1.016	> 3.0 g/dL	> 200 U/L	> 0.5	> 0.6

REPLACEMENT FLUIDS

	mEq/L						GLUCOSE
FLUID	Na	K	Cl	HCO$_3$	Ca	kcal/L	(g/L)
½ NS	77	-	77	-	-	-	-
NS	154	-	154	-	-	-	-
D5W	-	-	-	-	-	170	50
D10W	-	-	-	-	-	340	100
LR	130	4	109	28	3	9	-

NORMAL LAB VALUES*

ARTERIAL BLOOD GASES

pH	PaCO₂	PaO₂	HCO₃	Oxygen Saturation	Base Excess

| pH 7.35-7.45 | $PaCO_2$ 35-45 mm Hg | PaO_2 80-100 mm Hg | HCO_3 21-27 mEq/L | Oxygen Saturation 95-98% | Base Excess ± 2mEq/L |

URINE

Minimum Volume 0.5-1.0 mL/kg/hr
Specific Gravity 1.002-1.030
Osmolality 50-1400 mOsmol/kg
Creatinine, M 14-26, F 11-20 mg/kg/day
Creatinine Clearance
  M 90-136 mL/min/1.73 m²
  F 80-125 mL/min/1.73 m²
Urea Nitrogen 12-20 g/day

Sodium 40-220 mEq/day
Potassium 25-125 mEq/day
Calcium 100-300 mg/day
Phosphate 0.4-1.3 g/day
Uric Acid 250-750 mg/day

Amylase 1-17 U/hr
Glucose < 0.5 g/day
Albumin 10-100 mg/day
Protein 10-150 mg/day

5-HIAA 2-6 mg/day
17-Ketosteroids (17-KS)
  M 8-22, F 6-15 mg/day
17-Ketogenic Steroids (17-KGS)
  M 5-23, F 3-15 mg/day
17-Hydroxycorticosteroids (17-OHCS)
  M 3.0-10.0, F 2.0-8.0 mg/day
Homovanillic Acid (HVA) 1.4-8.8 mg/day
Metanephrine, total 0.05-1.2 µg/mg cre.

TOXICOLOGY

Acetaminophen, toxic > 200 µg/mL
COHgb, toxic > 20% saturation
Ethanol (mg/dL, non-alcoholic patient)
  > 100 intoxed, ataxic, slurred speech
  > 200 lethargic, stuporous, vomiting
  > 300 coma
  > 500 respiratory depression, death
Ethylene Glycol, toxic > 20 mg/dL
Lead, toxic > 100 µg/dL
Methanol, toxic > 200 mg/L
Salicylate, toxic > 300 µg/mL (trough)

CEREBROSPINAL FLUID

Pressure 70-180 mm CSF supine
WBC 0-5 mononuclear cells / µL
Protein 15-45 mg/dL
Glucose 40-70 mg/dL

SYNOVIAL FLUID

WBC < 200 /µL (<25% neutrophils)
  Trauma, OA, SLE < 3000 WBC/µL
  Gout, RA < 4000 WBC/µL
  Septic > 60000 WBC/µL
Protein ≤ 3.0 g/dL
Glucose > 40 mg/dL
Uric Acid < 8.0 mg/dL
LDH ≤ Serum LDH

ENDOCRINOLOGY

Aldosterone, supine 3-10 ng/dL,
  upright 5-30 ng/dL
Cortisol, 0800h 6-23, 1600h 3-15 µg/dL,
  2200h ≤ 50% of 0800h value
Estrogen, follicular 0-200, luteal
  160-400, menopausal ≤ 130 pg/mL
FSH, follicular 1-9, ovulation 6-26,
  luteal 1-9, menopausal 30-118 mU/mL
Gastrin < 100 pg/mL
Growth Hormone, M < 2, F < 10 ng/mL
  >60y, M < 10, F < 14 ng/mL
LH, follicular 1-12, midcycle 16-104,
  luteal 1-12, menopausal 16-66 mU/mL
Progesterone, follicular 0.15-0.7,
  luteal 2.0-25 ng/mL
Prolactin < 20 ng/mL
PTH 10-65 pg/mL
Testosterone, M, free 52-280 ng/mL,
  total 300-1000 ng/dL
T4, total 5.0-12.0 µg/dL
T4, free 0.8-2.3 ng/dL
T3, total 100-200 ng/dL
TBG 15-34 µg/dL
TSH < 10 µU/mL;
  >60y, M 2-7.3, F 2-16.8 µU/mL

*NOTE: Values given are for adults. Normal lab values vary between hospitals and laboratories. Check local normal values before instituting any treatment.

NORMAL LAB VALUES*

HEMATOLOGY

| WBC 4.5-11.0 x 10³ per µL | Hemoglobin M 13.5-17.5 g/dL F 12.0-16.0 g/dL | Platelets 150-450 x 10³ per µL |
| | Hematocrit M 39-49% F 35-45% | |

Neutrophils 57-67%
Segs 54-62%
Bands 3-5%
Lymphocytes 23-33%
Monocytes 3-7%
Eosinophils 1-3%
Basophils 0-1%

RBC, M 4.3-5.7, F 3.8-5.1 x 10⁶/µL
MCV 80-100 fL
MCH 26-34 pg/cell
MCHC 31-37% Hgb/cell
Reticulocyte Count 0.5-1.5%
Hemoglobin A1C 5.0-6.5%
Haptoglobin 26-185 mg/dL

PT 11-15 sec, aPTT 20-35 sec
Bleeding Time 2-7 min
Thrombin Time 6.3-11.1 sec
Fibrinogen 200-400 mg/dL
FDP < 10 µg/mL
ESR, M < 15, F < 20 mm/hr
D-Dimer ≤ 250 ng/mL DDU

CHEMISTRIES

| Sodium 135-145 mEq/L | Chloride 98-106 mEq/L | BUN 7-18 mg/dL | Glucose 70-115 mg/dL | Anion Gap 7-16 mEq/L |
| Potassium 3.5-5.1 mEq/L | Bicarbonate 22-29 mEq/L | Creatinine 0.6-1.2 mg/dL | | Osmolality 275-295 mOsm/kg |

Calcium, total 8.4-10.2 mg/dL
Calcium, ionized 4.65-5.28 mg/dL
Phosphate 2.7-4.5 mg/dL
>60y, M 2.3-3.7, F 2.8-4.1 mg/dL
Magnesium 1.3-2.1 mEq/L

Protein, total 6.0-8.0 g/dL
Albumin 3.5-5.5 g/dL
α₁-Fetoprotein < 10 ng/mL

Bilirubin, total 0.2-1.0 mg/dL
Bilirubin, conjugated 0-0.2 mg/dL

Lipase 10-140, >60y 18-180 U/L
Amylase 25-125 U/L
C-peptide 0.70-1.89 ng/mL
Total Cholesterol < 200 mg/dL
LDL Cholesterol < 130 mg/dL
HDL Cholest., M > 29, F > 35 mg/dL
Triglycrds., M 40-160, F 35-135 mg/dL

Lactate, venous 5.0-20.0 mg/dL
Uric Acid, M 3.5-7.2, F 2.6-6.0 mg/dL
Ammonia Nitrogen 10-50 µmol/L

Alk. Phos., M 38-126, F 70-230 U/L
LDH 90-190 U/L
Fraction 1, 18-33%; 2, 28-40%;
3, 18-30%; 4, 6-16%; 5, 2-13%
SGOT/AST and SGPT/ALT 7-40 U/L
GGT, M 9-50, F 8-40 U/L
CPK, M 38-174, F 26-140 U/L
CPK MB < 5%
Troponin T ≤ 0.01 ng/mL

Iron, M 65-175, F 50-170 µg/dL
TIBC 250-450 µg/dL
Iron Saturation, M 20-50, F 15-50%
Ferritin, M 20-250, F 10-120 µg/dL

Vitamin B12 100-700 pg/mL
Folate 3-16 ng/mL
Copper, M 70-140, F 80-155 µg/dL
Zinc 70-150 µg/dL

PSA < 4.0 ng/mL
Acid Phosphatase < 0.8 U/L
CEA < 2.5, smoker < 5.0 ng/mL
CA-125 < 35 U/mL

*NOTE: Values given are for adults. Normal lab values vary between hospitals and laboratories. Check local normal values before instituting any treatment.

NIH STROKE SCALE

1a. LEVEL OF CONSCIOUSNESS
0 = Alert
1 = Not alert but arousable
2 = Not alert and requires repeated stimulation
3 = Responds only with reflexes / autonomic effects or totally unresponsive

1b. LEVEL OF CONSCIOUSNESS QUESTIONS (ask month and age)
0 = Answers both questions correctly
1 = Answers one question correctly
2 = Answers neither question correctly

1c. LEVEL OF CONSCIOUSNESS COMMANDS (open/close eyes, grip/release hand)
0 = Performs both tasks correctly
1 = Performs one task correctly
2 = Performs neither task correctly

2. BEST GAZE
0 = Normal
1 = Partial gaze palsy, gaze abnormal in one or both eyes
2 = Forced deviation or total gaze paresis

3. VISUAL
0 = No visual loss
1 = Partial hemianopia
2 = Complete hemianopia
3 = Bilateral hemianopia (blind including cortical blindness)

4. FACIAL PALSY
0 = Normal symmetrical movements
1 = Minor paralysis
2 = Partial paralysis
3 = Complete paralysis

5. MOTOR ARM, 6. MOTOR LEG
0 = No drift
1 = Drift
2 = Some effort against gravity
3 = No effort against gravity
4 = No movement
UN = Amputation or joint fusion

7. LIMB ATAXIA
0 = Absent
1 = Present in one limb
2 = Present in two limbs
UN = Amputation or joint fusion

8. SENSORY
0 = Normal
1 = Mild-to-moderate sensory loss
2 = Severe to total sensory loss

9. BEST LANGUAGE
0 = Normal
1 = Mild-to-moderate aphasia
2 = Severe aphasia
3 = Mute, global aphasia

10. DYSARTHRIA
0 = Normal
1 = Mild-to-moderate dysarthria
2 = Severe dysarthria
UN = Intubated or other physical barrier

11. EXTINCTION AND INATTENTION
0 = No abnormality
1 = Visual, tactile, auditory, spatial, or personal inattention / extinction
2 = Profound hemi-inattention or extinction to more than one modality

NOTE: Scale used to measure neurological change in stroke patients.
See http://www.ninds.nih.gov/doctors/NIH_Stroke_Scale.pdf for full text.

ACLS SUSPECTED STROKE

Activate Emergency Response
ABCs, Vitals, Oxygen prn
IV, Labs, Check glucose and treat prn
Neurologic Screening Assessment
NIH Stroke / Canadian Neuro Scale

Activate Stroke Team
Time of Symptom Onset
H & P, Neurologic Exam
Emergent Brain CT or MRI
12-Lead ECG

CT SCAN WITH HEMORRHAGE
→ CONSULT NEUROLOGIST / NEUROSURGEON
Consider transfer if not available
Stroke or hemorrhage pathway

CT SCAN WITHOUT HEMORRHAGE
Check fibrinolytic exclusions
Repeat neuro exam - rapidly improving to normal?

FIBRINOLYTIC THERAPY CANDIDATE
Review risks / benefits with patient and family
→ rtPA
No anticoagulants or antiplatelet meds for 24 hrs.
Post rtPA stroke pathway, monitor BP, neurologic exam

NOT FIBRINOLYTIC THERAPY CANDIDATE
→ ASPIRIN
Stroke or hemorrhage pathway

ADMIT TO STROKE UNIT OR ICU

CANADIAN NEUROLOGICAL SCALE

MENTATION
Level Of Consciousness
Alert = 3.0
Drowsy = 1.5

Orientation
Oriented = 1.0
Disoriented or NA = 0

Speech
Normal = 1.0
Expressive Deficit = 0.5
Receptive Deficit = 0

COMPREHENSION DEFECT
Face Weakness
Symmetrical = 0.5
Asymmetrical = 0

Arms and Legs Weakness
Equal = 1.5
Unequal = 0

NO COMPREHENSION DEFECT
Face Weakness
None = 0.5
Present = 0

Proximal Arm Weakness
None = 1.5
Mild = 1.0
Significant = 0.5
Total = 0

Distal Arm Weakness
None = 1.5
Mild = 1.0
Significant = 0.5
Total = 0

Leg Weakness
None = 1.5
Mild = 1.0
Significant = 0.5
Total = 0

NOTE: Scale used to measure neurological change in stroke patients.
See http://stroke.ahajournals.org/content/17/4/731 for full text.

ACLS ADULT BRADYCARDIA WITH PULSE

Assess appropriateness for clinical condition
Heart rate typically < 50 beats per minute
Identify and treat underlying cause
Maintain airway, assist breathing as needed
O₂, pulse ox, BP, IV, cardiac monitor, 12-Lead ECG if available

PERSISTENT BRADYCARDIA Causing
Hypotension
Acutely altered mental status
Signs of shock
Ischemic chest discomfort
Acute heart failure

➜ **ATROPINE 0.5mg IV BOLUS**, q3-5 min to max total 3mg

➜ **TRANSCUTANEOUS PACING** or

➜ **DOPAMINE IV 2-10 mcg/kg/min** or

➜ **EPINEPHRINE IV 2-10 mcg/min**

Consider expert consultation
Consider transvenous pacing

ACLS ADULT TACHYCARDIA WITH PULSE

Assess appropriateness for clinical condition
Heart rate typically ≥150 beats per minute
Identify and treat underlying cause
Maintain airway, assist breathing as needed
O₂, pulse ox, BP, IV, cardiac monitor, 12-Lead ECG if available

PERSISTENT TACHYCARDIA Causing
Hypotension
Acutely altered mental status
Signs of shock
Ischemic chest discomfort
Acute heart failure

➜ **SYNCHRONIZED CARDIOVERSION**
Narrow regular: 50-100J
Narrow irregular: 120-200J biphasic or 200J monophasic
Wide regular: 100J
Wide irregular: defibrillation dose NOT synchronized

Consider sedation

IF REGULAR NARROW COMPLEX
Consider **ADENOSINE 6mg IV push**, second dose 12mg prn

WIDE QRS ≥ 0.12 SECOND
Consider **ADENOSINE 6mg IV push** if regular and monomorphic
Consider antiarrhythmic infusion (procainamide, amiodarone, sotalol)
Consider expert consultation

OTHERWISE
Vagal maneuvers
Adenosine (if regular), β-blocker or Ca⁺ channel blocker
Consider expert consultation

ACLS ACUTE CORONARY SYNDROMES

Symptoms suggestive of ischemia or infarction

IMMEDIATE E.D. TREATMENT
→ O_2 at 4L / minute and titrate if O_2 sat < 94%
→ ASPIRIN 160-325mg if not already given by EMS
→ NITROGLYCERIN SUBLINGUAL or SPRAY
→ MORPHINE IV if discomfort not relieved by nitroglycerin

CONCURRENT E.D. ASSESSMENT (<10 minutes)
VITALS, O_2 SAT, IV, TARGETED H&P
CHECK FIBRINOLYTIC CONTRAINDICATIONS
CARDIAC MARKER LEVELS, LYTES, COAGS
Portable **CHEST X-RAY** (<30 minutes)

ECG SUSPICIOUS ST ELEVATION OR NEW / PRESUMABLY NEW LBBB
ST-ELEVATION MI (STEMI)

Adjunctive therapies as indicated, do not delay reperfusion

TIME OF SYMPTOM ONSET ≤ 12 HOURS
FIBRINOLYSIS within 30 minutes of arrival
BALLOON INFLATION (PCI) within 90 minutes of arrival

TIME OF SYMPTOM ONSET > 12 HOURS
Go to ★ below

ECG SUSPICIOUS ST DEPRESSION OR DYNAMIC T-WAVE INVERSION
HIGH RISK UNSTABLE ANGINA / NON-ST-ELEVATION MI (UA / NSTEMI)

★ **TROPONIN ELEVATED OR HIGH-RISK PT** consider early invasive tx if:
Refractory ischemic chest discomfort Hemodynamic instability
Recurrent / persistent ST deviation   Signs of heart failure
Ventricular tachycardia

ADJUNCTIVE TREATMENTS AS INDICATED
Nitroglycerin
Heparin (UFH or LMWH)
Consider PO β-blockers, Clopidogrel, Glycoprotein IIb/IIIa inhibitor

✚ **ADMIT TO MONITORED BED, ASSESS RISK STATUS**
Continue ASA, heparin, other therapies as indicated
ACE inhibitor / ARB
HMG CoA reductase inhibitor (statin therapy)

ECG NORMAL / NONDIAGNOSTIC ST SEGMENT OR T WAVE CHANGES
LOW / INTERMEDIATE RISK ACS

Consider admission to E.D. chest pain unit or appropriate bed
Serial cardiac markers (including troponin) and ECG monitoring
Consider noninvasive diagnostic test

DEVELOPS ONE OR MORE GO TO ★ ABOVE
Clinical high-risk features
Dynamic ECG changes consistent with ischemia
Troponin elevated

ABNORMAL NONINVASIVE / PHYSIOLOGIC TESTING GO TO ✚ ABOVE

ACLS CARDIAC ARREST

CPR, OXYGEN, MONITOR / DEFIBRILLATOR

VENTRICULAR FIBRILLATION / VENTRICULAR TACHYCARDIA (VF/VT)

➔ **SHOCK**

➔ **CPR for 2 minutes**

IV / IO access

➔ **EPINEPHRINE 1 mg IV / IO** q3-5 minutes
(*OR* **VASOPRESSIN 40 U IV / IO** for 1st or 2nd epinephrine dose)

Consider advanced airway, capnography

➔ **AMIODARONE 300mg IV / IO**, second dose 150mg IV / IO

**RECHECK RHYTHM AND POSSIBLY SHOCK
AFTER EVERY 2 MINUTES OF CPR OR MEDICATION DOSE**

Treat reversible causes (see list below)

ASYSTOLE / PULSELESS ELECTRICAL ACTIVITY (PEA)

➔ **CPR for 2 minutes**

IV / IO access

➔ **EPINEPHRINE 1 mg IV / IO** q3-5 minutes
(*OR* **VASOPRESSIN 40 U IV / IO** for 1st or 2nd epinephrine dose)

Consider advanced airway, capnography

**RECHECK RHYTHM AND POSSIBLY SHOCK
AFTER EVERY 2 MINUTES OF CPR OR MEDICATION DOSE**

Treat reversible causes

Hypovolemia	Tension pneumothorax
Hypoxia	Tamponade (cardiac)
Hydrogen ion (acidosis)	Toxins
Hypo-/hyperkalemia	Thrombosis (pulmonary)
Hypothermia	Thrombosis (coronary)

ACLS IMMEDIATE POST CARDIAC ARREST CARE

Return Of Spontaneous Circulation (ROSC)

OPTIMIZE VENTILATION AND OXYGENATION
Maintain oxygen sat ≥ 94%
Consider advanced airway and waveform capnography
Do not hyperventilate

TREAT HYPOTENSION (SBP < 90 mm Hg)
IV / IO bolus 1-2 L normal saline or lactated Ringer's
Vasopressor infusion (epinephrine, dopamine, norepinephrine)
Treat reversible causes (see list above)
12-Lead ECG

DOES NOT FOLLOW COMMANDS: Consider induced hypothermia

STEMI or HIGH SUSPICION AMI: Coronary reperfusion

ADVANCED CRITICAL CARE

BLS HEALTHCARE PROVIDER

UNRESPONSIVE, NO NORMAL BREATHING
ACTIVATE EMERGENCY RESPONSE SYSTEM
GET AED / DEFIBRILLATOR

DEFINITE PULSE
  GIVE 1 BREATH EVERY 5-6 SEC
  CHECK PULSE every 2 minutes

NO PULSE
  BEGIN CPR 100 comp/min
  30 compressions / 2 breaths

AED / DEFIBRILLATOR ARRIVES

SHOCKABLE RHYTHM
  GIVE 1 SHOCK
  RESUME CPR for 2 minutes

NOT SHOCKABLE RHYTHM
  RESUME CPR for 2 minutes

RECHECK RHYTHM EVERY 2 MINUTES
Continue until ALS provider takes over or victim moves

NOTE: These are outlines of ACLS algorithms. Review complete ACLS algorithms by the AHA - www.heart.org - before instituting any treatment.

WAVEFORM MEASUREMENTS

P wave < 0.11 sec
PR interval 0.12-0.20 sec
QRS interval < 0.10 sec
QTc interval 0.33-0.47 sec

One Large Box 0.20 sec
One Small Box 0.04 sec

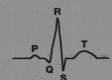

CARDIOPULMONARY VALUES

Central Venous 3-8 mm Hg
R. Atrium (mean) 0-8 mm Hg
R. Ventricle 15-30 / 0-8 mm Hg
Pulm. Artery 15-30 / 3-12 mm Hg
Pulm. Wedge (mean) 1-10 mm Hg
L. Ventricle 100-140 / 3-12 mm Hg
Aorta 100-140 / 60-90 mm Hg
Aa Gradient 5-15 mm Hg

Pulm. Resistance 20-130 d•s/cm^5
Syst. Resistance 700-1600 d•s/cm^5

Cardiac Output 3.5-7.5 L/min
Cardiac Index 2.5-3.5 L/min/m^2
Ejection Fraction 59-75%

Mitral Valve 4.0-6.0 cm^2
Aortic Valve 2.6-3.5 cm^2

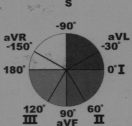

■ **LEFT AXIS DEVIATION**
■ **NORMAL AXIS**
■ **RIGHT AXIS DEVIATION**